MAITAKE
MUSHROOM &
D-FRACTION

The powerful healing abilities
of an ancient remedy

Shari Lieberman, Ph.D, CNS, FACN
AND **Ken Babal, C.N.**

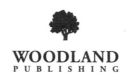

WOODLAND
P U B L I S H I N G

For order information or other inquiries, please contact us:
Woodland Publishing
P.O. Box 160
Pleasant Grove, Utah
84062
Visit us at our web site: www.woodlandpublishing.com
or call us toll-free: (800) 777-2665

The information in this book is for educational purposes only and is not recommended as a means of diagnosing or treating an illness. All matters concerning
physical and mental health should be supervised by a health practitioner knowl-
edgeable in treating that particular condition. Neither the publisher nor the
author directly or indirectly dispenses medical advice, nor do they prescribe any
remedies or assume any responsibility for those who choose to treat themselves.

ISBN 1-58054-344-8
Printed in the United States of America

Contents

Mushrooms: The Third Kingdom 5

A 50-Century Alliance 6

Nutritional Value of Mushrooms 6

Beta-Glucans and Cellular Immunity 7

    Adaptogenic and Tonifying Qualities 8

Maitake: King of Mushrooms 9

Cancer Research 10

    Maitake D-Fraction 10

    Immuno-Responses 11

    Tumor Inhibition 11

    Oral Absorption of D-Fraction 11

    Inhibition of Cancer Metastasis 11

    Anticarcinogenesis 12

    Enhancement of Chemotherapy 13

    Improving the Quality of Life For Cancer Patients 13

    Clinical Cases 15

    U.S. Cases 17

    Apoptosis and Prostate Cancer 18

    D-Fraction Approved by FDA for Study 19

Leading Practitioners Comment on Maitake 20

HIV and AIDS 21

    HIV Pioneers 21

Diabetes 22

High Blood Pressure 24
High Cholesterol and Triglycerides 25
Weight Control and Constipation 26
Syndrome X 26
Other Clinical Cases 27
How to Take Maitake 28
    Fresh or Dried Maitake 28
    Maitake Tablets 28
    The "One-and-Only" D-Fraction 29
    Teas 29
References 30

Mushrooms: The Third Kingdom

MUSHROOMS AND OTHER FUNGI have been called "the third king-dom." Being neither plant nor animal, they are a world unto them-selves. Their genetic make-up is actually closer to that of humans and animals than to plants. (We share approximately 30 percent of our DNA with mushrooms.) While plants absorb carbon dioxide and liberate oxygen, mushrooms mimic human respiration by cap-turing oxygen and exhaling carbon dioxide. But unlike humans who need light and fresh food, mushrooms feed on moist decaying, organic matter in deep shade. In our forests, mushrooms perform an essential ecological function of recycling leaves and dead plants. Mushrooms resemble plants in that they cannot move on their own and have cell walls. Yet mushrooms are not really plants as we gen-erally think of them. Instead of containing cellulose in their cell walls, they contain *chitin*, a substance also found in the exoskeleton of shellfish.

Many people feel uneasy when they learn that a mushroom is a fungus. The word "fungus" often brings to mind such unappealing pictures as athlete's foot, mildew in dirty shower stalls, moldy fruit and white fuzz on stale bread. In the U.S., mushrooms are often regarded with suspicion because of certain poisonous varieties. There is also the memory of the "magic mushrooms" of the 1960s which produced hallucinogenic trips similar to those of LSD. Even early cancer investigators were skeptical of purported benefits because mushrooms appeared to have properties similar to those of cancer—parasite- and fungus-like and fast-growing.

Mushrooms are just one of the many kinds of fungi. There are 100,000 species within the broad category of fungi, of which the penicillin mold is one, and there are 38,000 species of mushrooms.

Approximately fifty species of mushrooms are poisonous and another fifty demonstrate medicinal value, each with its own chemistry.

Mushrooms are among the largest organisms on the planet. Recently, a honey mushroom (*Armillaria ostoyae*) was discovered under 2,200 acres (about 3.5 square miles) of the Malheur National Forest in eastern Oregon. It eclipsed the previous record of a mushroom discovered in 1992 which covered a mere 1,500 acres in Washington state.

A 50-Century Alliance

Over thousands of years, mushrooms such as reishi, shiitake, maitake and others have been used to maintain and improve health, preserve youth and increase longevity. Reishi is among the top-ranked herbs in traditional Chinese medicine (TCM). Shiitake is also highly regarded and is said to boost "chi," or life-energy. In Japanese herbal medicine (called "kampo"), maitake is used as a treatment for a variety of conditions and as a tonic to strengthen the body and improve overall health. In ancient China and Japan, these mushrooms were so valued they were reserved only for emperors or royal families. The 5,300-year-old Ice Man, who was discovered in 1991 on the border or Austria and Italy, carried three kinds of mushrooms, suggesting that he considered them essential to his trek over the Alps.

Today, practitioners of TCM and kampo still regard medicinal mushrooms as the highest of tonics promoting overall well-being and vibrant health. In natural food and supplement stores, mushrooms are carving out their own niche as dietary supplements apart from herbs and vitamins.

Nutritional Value of Mushrooms

Many people mistakenly believe that mushrooms contribute little to health. Although specific nutritional content depends upon cultivation methods, mushrooms are generally rich sources of minerals, thiamin (B1), riboflavin (B2), and niacin (B3) as well as essential amino acids. Mushrooms also contain the provitamin ergosterol (vitamin D2) which is not found in vegetables. Ergosterol is converted to vitamin D in the body just as beta carotene in fruits and vegetables is converted to vitamin A. In addition, mushrooms are high in fiber while low in calories, making them the perfect dieting food.

Mushrooms have been valued throughout the world as both food and medicine. Approximately 700 species are used for food. Europeans and Asians have always appreciated the gastronomic value of wild mushrooms. In the United States, however, mushrooms are often underrated. Only recently have some of the more exotic varieties appeared in markets. Shiitake, portobello, enoki, oyster and porcini are now popular gourmet cuisine ingredients.

We are accustomed to hearing such phrases as "Milk—it does a body good" and "Orange juice—are you drinking enough?" Will we soon hear, "Have you had your mushrooms today?"

Beta-Glucans and Cellular Immunity

Just as there are many nutritional contributors to immunity, there are many aspects of immune function. In general, coordination among all glands and organs contributes to a strong and unified immune system. The most important immune function, however, occurs on a cellular level in the blood and tissues.

The lymphatic and circulatory systems are the "highways" for specialized white blood cells that travel throughout the body. White blood cells include B cells, T cells, natural killer cells and macrophages. Each have a different responsibility but all function together with the primary objective of recognizing, attacking and destroying bacteria, viruses, cancer cells and all substances seen as foreign. Without this coordinated effort we would not be able to survive more than a few days before succumbing to overwhelming infection.

Infection sets off "alarms" that alert the immune system to bring out its defensive weapons. Natural killer cells and the "Pacman-like" macrophages rush to the scene to gobble up and digest infected cells. If this first line of defense fails to control the threat, antibodies, produced by B cells upon the order of helper T cells, are custom-designed to hone in on the invader.

In addition to essential nutrients, mushrooms contain many semi-essential, non-vitamin factors that have protective and therapeutic value against certain diseases. One of these compounds is beta-glucan, a complex carbohydrate or polysaccharide composed of glucose sugar molecules strung together. Scientific studies show that beta-glucan is largely responsible for the immune-activating and anti-tumor properties of maitake and some other medicinal mushrooms.[1]

Although we generally think of carbohydrates as providing energy to body cells, research reveals that many are involved in molecular recognition. Specifically, cell-surface carbohydrates help to facilitate communication between cells in certain kinds of interactions. Receptors for beta-glucans can be found on macrophages, the large white blood cells that engage in phagocytosis, the swallowing of microorganisms, pathogens and tumor cells. When macrophages are activated, they in turn trigger a cascade of immune-stimulating events.

Beta-glucans are found in other superfoods, including oats, yeast and other medicinal mushrooms. However, the chemical structure of maitake beta-glucan (1,6 beta-glucan carrying branched chains of 1,3 beta-glucan) is unique due to its greater degree of molecular branching.

ADAPTOGENIC AND TONIFYING QUALITIES

Ancient oriental medicine did not have knowledge of beta-glucans or cellular immunity but understood that health depends upon the body's capacity to maintain equilibrium (yin/yang balance) by adapting to changing conditions. Maitake and other medicinal mushrooms are beneficial to this process because they are adaptogenic and tonifying. Adaptogens are defined as substances that help adjust altered/stressed body conditions back to normal. In other words, adaptogens can help individuals maintain healthy levels of blood pressure, blood sugar, cholesterol and body weight. Similarly, a tonic is a substance that strengthens or invigorates organs or the entire organism.

In TCM (traditional Chinese medicine), mushrooms are used to balance the effects of excessive meat-eating by neutralizing toxic residues. Maitake, said to be the most cleansing of the mushrooms, targets the liver and lungs. Health practitioners know that if liver function can be improved, overall health will benefit because the liver is the largest organ within the body and performs innumerable functions including detoxification of internally and externally produced poisons.

Maitake: King of Mushrooms

The scientific name for maitake, *Grifola frondosa*, is derived from the common name of a mushroom in Italy and refers to a mythical beast which is half-lion and half-eagle. Maitake is indigenous to the northeastern part of Japan. The mushroom has a rippling appearance with no caps and grows in clusters at the foot of oak trees. To the Japanese, this conveys an image of dancing butterflies, thus the name maitake (pronounced *my TAH keh*), literally "dancing mushroom." Others say that maitake is so named because people who found it deep in the mountains would begin dancing with joy because of its delicious taste and wonderful health benefits. During the feudal era of Japan, maitake also had monetary value and was exchanged for the same weight in silver by local lords who in turn offered it to the national leader, the shogun.

Maitake has other unique characteristics. It is the only edible mushroom in the Monkey's Bench family, which are well-known immune enhancers. Maitake is a giant, often reaching twenty inches at the base. A single cluster can weigh as much as 100 pounds. Its large size and amazing health benefits are why it has come to be called "the king of mushrooms."

Cancer Research

MAITAKE D-FRACTION

Most immune-potentiating and anticancer research favors maitake "D-fraction," the protein-bound form of beta glucan extracted from the mushroom and developed by Maitake Products, Inc., a pioneer of mushroom products in the U.S. It should be noted that all study reports introduced herein have been based on its product under the brand name of Grifron D-Fraction.

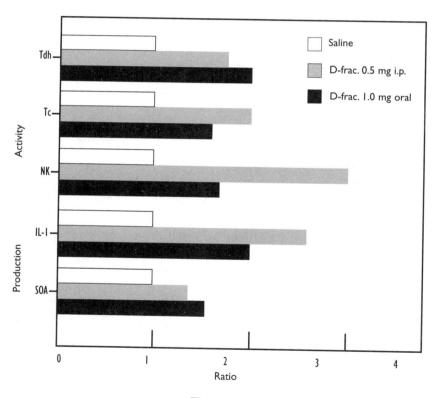

Figure 1.
Immuno-responses by maitake. It acts to potentiate cellular immune-competent cells, where macrophage, NK, LAK, Tc and Tdh cells are activated by D-fraction.

IMMUNO-RESPONSES

Maitake D-fraction shows an immune-activating and anti-tumor effect in tumor-bearing mice.[2] Unlike chemotherapeutic drugs, maitake does not kill cancer cells directly but activates the body's immune cells. Figure 1 shows how much each type of immune-competent cell is activated by maitake D-fraction. Activity of natural killer (NK) cells and cytotoxic T cells (Tc) was increased from 1.5 to 3.0 times by oral administration or injection. Also seen was an increase of production of interleukin-1 (IL-1), which activates T cells, and superoxide anions (SOA), which damage tumor cells. In other words, maitake D-fraction not only activates various effector cells to attack tumor cells, but also potentiates the activities of various mediators.

TUMOR INHIBITION

Research shows that maitake is surprisingly potent and far superior to lentinan (shiitake), PSK (kawaratake) and reishi (mannentake) in terms of breast tumor growth inhibition (Table 1.).[3] PSK is the world's best-selling cancer drug (sold in Europe and Japan) but was not effective in this study. The Japan Health and Welfare Ministry instructs doctors to use PSK only in combination with other chemotherapeutic agents.

ORAL ABSORPTION OF D-FRACTION

Many anticancer drugs are only effective by injection. Maitake has the advantage of being effective when taken orally. D-fraction has been confirmed to be the optimal choice for oral administration and demonstrates the same effectiveness (or better) as an injection.[4] Table 2 compares the effect of D-fraction oral administration versus injection on skin and breast tumors in mice.

INHIBITION OF CANCER METASTASIS

Preventing the spread, or metastasis, of cancer from one area of the body to another is a major concern in cancer treatment since it

Group of Mice	Dosage	Inhibition Ratio
Control		0%
Maitake extract (D-fraction)	0.5 mg/kg wgt. 1.0 mg	86.0% 86.6%
Lentinan (shiitake)	1.0 mg	54.4%
PSK (kawaratake)	30.0 mg	-7.1%
Reishi (mannetake)	1.0 mg 50.0 mg	5.2% 36.8%

Table 1.
Tumor growth inhibition in intraperitoneal injection of
mushroom extracts (against sarcoma 180 tumor)

Mice	Tumor System	Growth Inhibition	
		Oral Admin.	Intraperitoneal
C3H	MM-46 carcinoma (breast)	64.0% (1.5 mg)	83.2% (1.0 mg)
CDFI	IMC carcinoma (skin)	75% (1.5 mg)	47.7% (1.0 mg)
C57BL/6	B-16 melanoma (skin)	27.3% (1.5 mg)	25.6% (1.0 mg)

Table 2.
Comparison of tumor growth inhibition after oral and
intraperitoneal administration

can have catastrophic results. A study was designed to see if maitake could inhibit metastasis. Mice were injected with cancer cells and then divided into three groups and fed (A) a control (normal) diet; (B) a diet consisting of 20 percent maitake powder; or (C) a control diet, but with additional injections of one milligram per kilogram of body weight of D-fraction.[5]

It was found that metastasis was inhibited by 81.3 percent in the maitake-fed group and by 91.3 percent in the group injected with D-fraction, while there was no inhibition whatever in the group receiving the regular diet.

ANTICARCINOGENESIS

Researchers also wanted to determine if maitake could prevent cancer from developing in normal cells. Three groups of mice were fed (A) a control diet, (B) a diet containing 20 percent maitake powder or (C) oral administration of 1 mg/kg body weight of D-fraction thirty times.[6] The mice were then given a carcinogenic (cancer-causing) chemical three times at seven-day intervals.

After sixty days, the tumors that developed in the liver were counted. The occurrence rate of liver cancer in the D-fraction group (C) and the 20 percent maitake-fed group (B) were 9.7 percent and 22.2 percent respectively while that of the control group (A) was 100 percent. The results of this study suggest that maitake may be helpful in reducing cancer risk from the numerous chemical carcinogens in our environment.

ENHANCEMENT OF CHEMOTHERAPY

One study compared D-fraction with mitomycin-C (MMC), one of the strongest and widely-used chemotherapeutic drugs having very severe side effects as well.[7] With just a small dose, the maitake extract produced approximately an 80 percent shrinkage in tumors in mice compared to 45 percent with MMC. When the two agents were combined in half-doses, an astonishing 98 percent shrinkage was achieved in fourteen days demonstrating an apparent synergy between the two agents.

IMPROVING THE QUALITY OF LIFE FOR PATIENTS

Figure 2 shows the results of a nonrandomized human study of the efficacy of maitake against various advanced cancers presented at the Adjuvant Nutrition in Cancer Treatment Symposium in Tampa, Florida in October 1995.[8] The 165 patients who participated in the study were between the ages of twenty-five and sixty-five and were diagnosed with stage III–IV cancer (advanced cancer). They were given maitake D-fraction 35–100 mg (equivalent to about 35–100 drops) per day along with maitake tablets only, or D-fraction accompanied by chemotherapy.

Tumor regression or significant symptom improvements were observed among 11 of 15 breast cancer patients, 12 of 18 lung cancer patients and 7 out of 15 liver cancer patients. If taken with chemotherapy, these response rates improved by 12 to 18 percent.

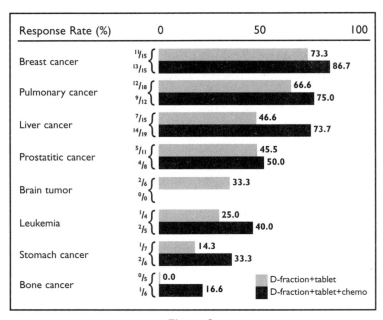

Figure 2.
Summary of trial results against various cancers

A number of patients were diagnosed as stage I after previously being diagnosed as stage III. Also, some drastic remissions were seen. An egg-sized brain tumor in a 44-year-old male completely disappeared after taking maitake D-fraction for four months. (See "Clinical Cases.") Most patients taking maitake claimed improvement of overall symptoms even when tumor regression was not observed. Although this was not a blind, placebo-controlled study, results suggest that breast, lung and liver cancers are more favorably affected by maitake treatment than cancer of the bone, stomach or blood (leukemia). This study also demonstrates that maitake has a synergistic effect with chemotherapy. In some cases, maitake treatment alone was almost effective as combination therapy.

It is important to note that many severe side effects of chemotherapy for all types of cancer were ameliorated when maitake was included with conventional treatment. Symptoms of nausea, hair-loss and leukopenia (deficiency of white blood cells) were alleviated in 90 percent of patients. Reduction of pain was also reported by 83 percent of patients. Authors of the study conclude that maitake improves the immune system and helps to maintain quality of life for patients resulting in possible remission of cancer without side effects.

CLINICAL CASES

Here are some typical clinical cases presented at the above symposium, showing improvement by oral administration of maitake D-fraction and tablets:

(1) Male, age 51, stage III liver cancer

The patient had received Adriamycin (ADM) since 1993, but refused it because of insufficient effectiveness and severe side effects. He has been taking 35 mg of D-fraction and 4 g of maitake tablets per day. Eight months later, bilirubin and albumin levels are improved. Bilirubin reduced to 1.8 mg/dl from 4.7 mg/dl. Albumin improved from 2.1 g/dl to 3.7 g/dl and prothrombin activation was increased to 92 percent from 36 percent. Because of tumor regression, his doctor reclassified him from stage III to stage II.

(2) Female, age 56, stage III liver cancer

This patient was diagnosed in stage III with serum bilirubin of 3.5 mg/dl, albumin of 2.8 g/dl and prothrombin activation of 48 percent. Diameter of tumor was more than 2 cm and metastases to lymph nodes were observed. She received transcatheter arterial embolization (TAE) in January 1994, and was then administered chemotherapeutic drugs such as ADM, Cisplatin (CDDP) and 5-FU, but she did not show any improvement. In December 1994, she started taking 55 mg (approximately 55 drops) of D-fraction and 6 g of maitake tablets every day. As of July 1995, her value of bilirubin was 2.7, albumin 3.1 and prothrombin activation 63 percent. She improved tremendously and was reclassified as stage I.

(3) Female, age 53, stage III lung cancer

In November 1993, this patient was diagnosed as stage III-A. Chemotherapeutic drugs CDDP 80 mg/m, CPA 350 mg/m and

ADM 50 mg/m2 were administered. However, she gave up taking them in March 1994 because of severe side effects. Since then she has switched to taking 50 mg (50 drops) D-fraction and 4 g of tablets. After fourteen months, she also improved and was upgraded to stage I.

(4) Male, age 71, stage IV lung cancer

Patient was diagnosed as advanced stage IV and told by his doctors that he had three months to live at most. He could not take chemotherapeutics, but he could take 70 mg (70 drops) of D-fraction and 9 g of tablets every day. Unfortunately, he died twenty months later. However, tumor size was reduced and the overall symptoms improved, being diagnosed as stage III-A before his death. Tumors that had metastasized in remote areas disappeared. He did not claim to feel much pain. Though he died, it appears that maitake contributed to extending his life for seventeen months beyond his doctors' estimate.

(5) Female, age 45, breast cancer

ER+ (estrogen receptor positive) was observed on this patient, who had 1.8 cm diameter of tumor. In April 1992, she underwent surgical removal of one breast. She then received chemotherapy including 5-FU and ADM until February 1994, but cancer recurrence (diameter 0.9 cm) was found in April 1994. She refused to take surgery this time and started taking 100 mg (about 100 drops) D-fraction and 5 g maitake tablets every day. After six months, the dose of D-fraction was reduced to 50 mg a day. In May 1995, complete regression of the recurred tumor was confirmed by her physician.

(6) Male, age 44, brain tumor

This is an example of D-fraction working very well. The patient has taken 100 mg (about 100 drops) D-fraction and 6 g maitake tablets every day for four months without taking any other medication, including chemotherapy and radiation. He had received chemotherapy (Lomustine: CCNU) 135 mg for four cycles beginning in February 1994. Because of severe side effects, no treatment was given for four months before starting maitake administration.

After four months, the chicken egg-sized brain tumor was confirmed by MRI to have completely disappeared.

U.S. CASES

Some practitioners in the United States also confirmed the effectiveness of maitake D-fraction in brain tumor patients, though not as dramatically as in clinical case #6 (on previous page). Robert Murphy, N.D., of Connecticut has used maitake D-fraction on his patients and has seen improvements in brain tumors:

"I had agreed to do an uncontrolled in-office study of administering maitake D-fraction 200 mg twice a day to a 44-year-old patient with mucinous adenocarcinoma of the brain. He had been given this diagnosis in May, 1994 and it was also revealed that he had a tumor in the proximal left femur. He was initially treated with Decadion to reduce brain edema and whole brain radiation. I phoned this gentleman in November and he was feeling well and had a repeat MRI done in October which demonstrated significant improvement and reduction of tumor size . . . maitake may well have played a part in this. Therefore, I would recommend he continue on maitake D-fraction."

In a report published in *Alternative Therapies* (May/June 2001), Eric Scheinbart, M.D., of Savannah, Georgia relates a case history of a 56-year-old patient with multiple myeloma and antibiotic-resistant pneumonia. Multiple myeloma is characterized by infiltration of bone by malignant cells that form tumors and fractures. The condition is usually progressive and fatal. The patient had underwent three unsuccessful bone marrow transplantations following three whole-body irradiations. Despite transfusions, his red blood cell and platelet counts continued to decline as did his kidney function. Fifteen months later he was admitted to the hospital for pneumonia which was determined to be Vancomycin-resistant. At this point, he was instructed to go home and "get his affairs in order."

On his family's urging, he decided to try an alternative therapy. He was put on maitake D-fraction liquid (2 droppers-full, three times a day) along with Ayurvedic herbs, thymic protein and nutritional supplements. Within one week he was feeling better and was ambulatory. Two months later, he was pronounced "miraculously in remission and without pneumonia." Two years after initial diagnosis, the patient recently returned from a cruise and was playing golf.

APOPTOSIS AND PROSTATE CANCER

Now at the forefront of cancer research is the study of apoptosis. Apoptosis is cell death programmed by a specific set of so-called suicide genes. Scientists have discovered that all cells, including cancer cells, have this potential to self-destruct. They are interested in finding substances that induce this biochemical reaction.

Recently, researchers at New York Medical College found that maitake D-fraction has apoptosis-inducing activity against prostate

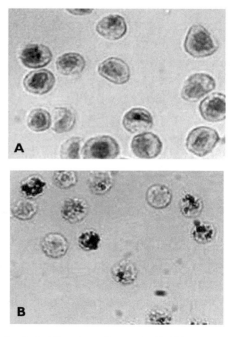

Figure 3. In situ hybridization. Control cells (A) were not treated with D-fraction, whereas cells treated with D-fraction (B) resulted in cell apoptosis. ("Induction of Apoptosis in Human Prostatic Cancer Cells with Beta-Glucan," Drs. Tazaki and Konno, Molecular Urology, Vol. 4, No. 1, 2000.)

cells in vitro.[9] When prostate cancer cells were treated with D-fraction, almost complete cell death was observed in twenty-four hours.

In addition, similar studies were conducted on prostate cancer cells using other natural extracts from hime-matsutake mushroom, reishi and kelps, which are well-known as natural antitumor agents in Japan. However, both hime-matsutake and kelps were essentially ineffective while reishi extract induced a greater than 50 percent cancer-cell death, which is much less potent compared to the greater than 95 percent cancer-cell death achieved by maitake D-fraction.

When maitake D-fraction was combined with vitamin C, there was a synergistic effect. As little as 1/16 to 1/8 of the original maitake dose combined with vitamin C was found to be nearly as effective as the maitake dose alone. These results suggest that, among the natural extracts tested thus far, the D-fraction appears to have the most profound cytotoxic effect on prostatic cancer cells and that, when combined with vitamin C, a synergistic effect is observed.

D-FRACTION APPROVED BY FDA FOR STUDY

In 1998, the Food and Drug Administration (FDA) approved an Investigational New Drug (IND) application from Maitake Products, Inc. of New Jersey[10] to conduct phase II clinical trials using maitake D-fraction on advanced breast- and prostate-cancer patients. In consideration of previous maitake research, the FDA authorized skipping a usual first phase toxicity study, going directly to the second phase. The ongoing study will examine the immune-activating effect of maitake on tumor size, clinical symptoms and quality of life.

Although not the first study of a natural substance for use in medicine, it is one of only a few, with just one or two known ever to have been FDA-approved. Without the FDA seal of approval, D-fraction cannot be marketed as a cancer treatment, tumor reductor or inhibitor. "The FDA study is a necessary first step to convince a skeptical American public and medical profession that nature provides the key to good health and without the potential toxic side effects often associated with chemically-produced medicines" says Mike Shirota, CEO and founder of Maitake Products, Inc. "D-fraction will ultimately be found beneficial in other cancers and diseases such as AIDS and chronic fatigue. Nutraceuticals, as opposed to pharmaceuticals, will lead the way to an enlightened new century."

Leading Practitioners Comment on Maitake

In the June 1994 issue of his newsletter, *Health Revelations*, Robert Atkins, M.D., wrote "Ralph Moss, author of several excellent books on cancer and alternative therapies, has researched more than 100 natural, effective cancer therapies. You'd think that he'd have a tough time identifying the most promising one, but when I asked him to do just that, he replied with just two words: medicinal mushrooms."

In his July 1996 issue, Dr. Atkins noted: "Some two years have passed since I last wrote about what may be the best of cancer antagonists, maitake mushrooms. Since then, some significant scientific advances have elevated the fungus even higher on my list of safe anti-cancer agents."

Andrew Weil, M.D., a prominent figure in the field of alternative/complimentary medicine, praised the "king of mushrooms" in an article in *Natural Health* (May/June 1993): "Research on the therapeutic properties of maitake is better and more extensive than that on other species . . . this mushroom is delicious." In his book *8 Weeks to Optimum Health*, he states, "My tonic of choice at the moment is an extract called maitake D-fraction, which concentrates the immune-boosting constituents . . . and since I've been using it I almost never get colds."

In a seminar called "Cancer: A Holistic Approach," presented at the Natural Products Expo West in Los Angeles (March 8-11, 2001), Mark Kaylor, an herbalist based in Costa Mesa, California, stated, "One remedy I use across the board is maitake mushroom. In my opinion, it is the strongest immune-modulator we have available to us, particularly for these chronic immune disorders. I've used it now for about seven years. My youngest client that used it was four years old. My oldest is now seventy-six, so it is a very safe substance."

HIV and AIDS

Maitake's anti-HIV properties have been recognized in both Japan and the U.S. The National Cancer Institute (NCI) confirmed the efficacy of D-fraction against HIV early in 1992, one year after the National Institute of Health (Japan) announced the same conclusion.[11] This result indicated that D-fraction can prevent HIV-infected helper T-cells from being destroyed by as much as 97 percent in vitro. This is very important because measuring a patient's helper T-cell count is considered as a benchmark in monitoring the progression of HIV to full-blown AIDS. Moreover, the researchers at NCI admitted that the maitake extract is as powerful as AZT (a commonly prescribed drug for AIDS, and the only FDA-approved drug at the time) but without toxic side effects associated with AZT. These prestigious research institutes confirmed in test-tube experiments that D-fraction enhances the activity of other immune cells as well as T lymphocytes. Since then, a number of practitioners involved in AIDS/HIV treatment have reported favorable responses in patients, including increases in helper T-cells and reversal of HIV-positive status to HIV-negative. This feedback supports what the studies show. Some physicians are also applying D-fraction extract topically as a treatment for Kaposi's sarcoma, a skin cancer which often develops in AIDS patients.

HIV PIONEERS

The pioneers who developed such treatments are two American AIDS researchers: Dr. Joan Priestley (Omni Medical Center, Anchorage, Alsaska) and Dr. David Hughes (Hyperbaric Oxygen Institute, San Bernardino, California). Dr. Priestley has found considerable improvement in her HIV/AIDS patients taking maitake. She has found that her patients' T-lymphocyte cell counts have stabilized or increased over the course of treatment. She has also found D-fraction to be a more effective treatment than maitake tablets alone. She states, "I have used maitake products on my patients for some time now and have been very impressed with the results. Topical application produced good regression of Kaposi's sarcoma lesions in one AIDS patient, a major accomplishment."

One of Dr. David Hughes' patients has claimed that his HIV-positive status was turned to negative by his use of maitake. On July 14, 1994, he tested positive for HIV, but a follow-up test result dated August 23 showed HIV-negative.

Dr. Hughes has focused his research on treating Kaposi's sarcoma, an often fatal skin condition that effects 40 percent of HIV/AIDS patients. According to Dr. Hughes, maitake D-fraction may be applied directly to the Kaposi's sarcoma lesions. He reports that lesions have disappeared within several days. Dr. Hughes recommends the following treatment:

Take two-thirds maitake D-fraction liquid extract plus one-third DMSO (dimethylsulfoxide). Apply this mixture with Q-tip to the Kaposi's sarcoma lesions. The lesions reduce in a few days. Dr. Hughes has added two cautions, however. The mix gets quite hot— so it seems that maitake will react chemcially with DMSO. Also, some patients who kept using it continuously got quite "high." We therefore tell patients not to use it more than four times per day.

Diabetes

Diabetes affects 16 million Americans, of whom approximately 95 percent are non-insulin dependent (Type II). Diabetes can cause death and is a risk factor for other diseases, including atherosclerosis, kidney disease and loss of nerve function.

Maitake has been confirmed to contain substances with anti-diabetic activity. Recent studies indicate that maitake can control blood glucose levels by reducing insulin resistance and enhancing insulin sensitivity. The results of a test on mice that have an obesity gene and are genetically diabetic were impressive.[12] On a regular diet, the blood glucose level and body weight of these mice increases with age. However, if maitake is mixed with the feed (20 percent) biomarkers such as blood glucose, insulin and triglycerides and body weight are maintained at a significantly lower level than controls. The glucose level of the maitake-feed group was 200 mg/dl after an eight-week period, showing little change from the start of the experiment, while the level of mice in the control group on normal feed rose to 400 mg/dl. Insulin and triglyceride levels were also significantly lowered, increasing only to 1/3 to 1/2 that of controls. Triglyceride levels in controls increased to 780 mg/dl (doubled) while that of the maitake-feed group remained virtually unchanged. Also, body weights of the maitake-feed group were lighter than those of the control group.

Following this test, a crossover test was also conducted in which the feed was altered at the beginning of the fifth week. At this point, maitake-feed was fed to the control group and normal-feed was given to the maitake-feed group. Blood glucose of mice in the control group, which had risen to 400 mg/dl, decreased to 230 mg/dl the week after administration of the maitake feed began. After two weeks, it decreased further to 155 mg/dl, which was below the start-up, pre-treatment level. The levels of insulin and triglycerides demonstrated similar changes as the group's diet was altered from normal feed to maitake feed. Researchers concluded that the changes in glucose values were caused by the administration of the maitake feed prior to the change in body weight and that maitake is effective in reducing glucose levels, insulin resistance and triglycerides in diabetic mice.

Another study indicates the anti-diabetic activity of maitake is related to metabolism of absorbed glucose rather than an inhibition of enzymes or glucose absorption at the intestinal mucosa.[13] It is interesting that some studies indicate an immunological/viral disorder as the basis for insulin- and non-insulin-dependent diabetes. In other words, a weakened immune system contributes to elevated blood glucose levels, which further weakens the immune system. Maitake's immuno-potentiating qualities may be part of the mechanism that helps to maintain healthy blood sugar levels.

As mentioned previously, maitake is free from the side effects often associated with conventional drug treatment. Maitake will not affect blood sugar levels in patients without diabetes.

Overall, it appears that maitake may play a role in effectively treating diabetes and related disorders, such as Syndrome X.

High Blood Pressure

Administration of maitake to hypertensive rats has been studied.[14] When fed maitake, blood pressure was reduced by 50 mmgHg compared to controls on a regular diet after four days. Further, a one-time feeding of an ether-soluble extract of maitake showed a remarkable result. In just four hours, blood pressure was lowered from 200 mmgHg to 115.

Abram Ber, M.D., of Scottsdale, Arizona, treated over thirty patients with maitake during a period of two to three months. He states, "When on medication, the blood pressure is all over the place, but with maitake mushroom there is a gradual decrease in blood pressure toward normalcy. Further, there are absolutely no side effects." Dr. Ber's treatment program includes three grams of whole dried maitake tablets per day for the first week, four grams per day for the second week, then five grams per day as blood pressure indicates. "Sometimes," he says, "blood pressure is dose-related."

Scott Gerson, M.D., Director of the Foundation for Holistic Medical Research in New york City, has also conducted studies on maitake's effectiveness in lowering blood pressure.

Eleven patients (seven men and four women) between forty-six and forty-eight years old with "documented essential hypertension" were studied. All eleven subjects were instructed to take three 500 mg caplets of maitake mushroom (Grifron) twice per day in the morning and evening at least ninety minutes away from food. Blood pressure was then measured weekly in the same clinical setting for an average of six weeks. There was a mean decrease in systolic BP of about 14 mmHg and a mean decrease in diastolic BP of about 8 mmHg. It is notable that there were no adverse effects reported by any of the subjects. In fact, all of the subjects reported feeling quite well during the study.

Dr. Gerson concluded that "I was left with a strong suspicion that maitake does indeed reduce blood pressure in hypertensive patients."

Michael Williams, M.D., Ph.D., Chief Medical Officer of Cancer Treatment Centers of America, shared his own experience of maitake's blood pressure-lowering activity:

"I am six feet tall with a family history of hypertension, with blood pressure ranging from 150/105 to 140/90. Systolic blood pressure before and one hour after one, two or four maitake pills ranged from 136 to 124, from 140 to 128, and from 146 to 134 on different test days. Diastolic blood pressures remained 88–92. The 8–12 percent decrease in systolic pressure was maintained for up to six hours. I resumed taking ten to twelve maitake pills in divided dose throughout the day. Blood pressures have remained at or below 120/80 for over two months without Vasotec [a prescription drug for hypertension]."

Dr. Williams cautioned, however, to avoid large doses on an empty stomach with beer. This may cause some severe hypotensive (low blood pressure) responses.

It should be pointed out that for lowering high blood pressure, practitioners use whole maitake mushroom tablets containing all fractions, rather than D-fraction.

High Cholesterol and Triglycerides

One of the chief causes of death and disability among elderly people is atherosclerosis. There is no doubt that the high-calorie and high-cholesterol American diet has contributed heavily to the incidence of serious degenerative diseases such as stroke and heart attack. Also, the lipid compounds called triglycerides are known to be strongly associated with cardiovascular disease, especially in older women.

In an animal test using rats which were fed (1) a regular diet, (2) one containing 5 percent shiitake or (3) one containing 5 percent maitake, the maitake-fed group experienced greater reduction of blood and liver cholesterol and triglyceride levels than the shiitake-fed group or the normal-fed group.[15] This suggests that maitake may have cardioprotective effects and reduce the risk of stroke and cardiovascular disease.

Weight Control and Constipation

Maitake is high in dietary fiber, an important component of a healthful diet. Fiber helps to prevent constipation by holding moisture in the bowel and increasing peristaltic action. Animal data show that the water content of the stool is significantly increased after feeding with maitake powder.

Maitake's anti-obesity activity has been studied in both animals and humans.[16] The results of tests with overweight rats indicate that after eighteen weeks those fed unheated maitake powder lost weight, whereas controls gained weight.

In a human study conducted by M. Yokota, M.D., at the Koseikai Clinic in Tokyo, patients lost weight on maitake.[17] Thirty patients were given twenty 500-mg tablets of maitake powder daily for a period of two months with no change in their regular diets. All of the patients lost weight (between seven and twenty-six pounds) with an average loss of eleven to thirteen pounds. Dr. Yokota surmises that the patients would have continued to lose weight if they had continued the program beyond the two months.

Syndrome X

Maitake has been shown to be beneficial for various disorders that can be grouped as conditions of excess, including one or more of the following: high blood levels of glucose, cholesterol, triglycerides, and insulin, as well as elevation in blood pressure and body weight. Today, scientists have coined a term for this cluster of symptoms which often occurs in older Americans, calling it "Syndrome X." Recently, Syndrome X has entered public consciousness through several best-selling books.

At Georgetown University, Harry Preuss, M.D., has conducted research to isolate other fractions in maitake that are responsible for its anti-hypertensive and anti-diabetic action.[18] Dr. Preuss believes that the various compounds in maitake influence the glucose/insulin system favorably and help to prevent the onset of age-related chronic disorders known as Syndrome X.

Other Clinical Cases

Abram Ber, M.D., is a long-time user of maitake mushroom products for a number of conditions. Dr. Ber gave six patients with uterine fibroids maitake tablets and found substantial reduction of fibroids six months to one year after beginning maitake treatment.[19] The patients conditions improved to a point at which surgery was usually not indicated. In general, Dr. Ber's treatment program is two tablets three times per day (three grams) and up to eight grams, depending on the size of the individual.

According to Dr. Ber, at least twelve patients with prostatic cancer have been treated with maitake tablets, resulting in amelioration of symptoms. In particular, there was improvement in urinary flow as well as frequency.

Another long-time user of maitake is Peter D'Adamo, N.D., of Greenwich, Connecticut, author of the best-selling *Eat Right for Your Type* (G.P. Putnam's Sons, 1996). He writes, "My observations cause me to feel very strongly that maitake mushroom and D-fraction accelerate the rate of healing and also have a complementary effect with other remedies that I use. One good case was a leukemia patient who had received chemotherapy. The tumor had metastasized to her spleen during the year after the treatment. The tumor grew fast and her spleen was swollen when she came to me. I gave her D-fraction and instructed her to take a half teaspoon twice a day. After a while, the tumor completely disappeared." He added that this was not a particularly rare case.

In 1993, Dr. D'Adamo treated thirty to thirty-five cancer patients and about fifteen HIV-positive patients, using primarily maitake mushroom in conjunction with a few other natural remedies. He has successfully used maitake in treating prostate cancer in men whose previous chemotherapy had been unsuccessful. He has used it successfully in treating pulmonary metastasis (the spreading of cancer through the circulatory system). These results were confirmed by physicians in Massachusetts General Hospital using CAT scans and magnetic imaging. He has successfully used maitake mushrooms in treating other cancer as well, including those of the liver, breast and colon. Dr. D'Adamo also theorizes that maitake has a potentiating effect on shark cartilage supplements in inhibiting angiogenesis (growth of new blood vessels that feed tumors).

How To Take Maitake

FRESH OR DRIED MAITAKE

Fresh mushrooms can be simmered, stuffed, sauteed, grilled and broiled. Dried mushrooms need to be soaked in water until soft before adding to soups, stews, sauces and stir fry.

Here are a few tips for preparing fresh and dried maitake that help to minimize nutrient losses. The D-fraction (beta-glucan extract), which activates the immune system, is hot water extractable. That is, it dissolves in the cooking water. As with cooking vegetables, you must recover the liquid to make use of all nutrients. The water in which maitake has been steamed, soaked or boiled can be used for soups, stews or sauces. Other compounds in maitake that are critical for lowering high blood pressure, high blood sugar and high cholesterol could be fat-soluble. This means that if you stir-fry, these substances will dissolve into the cooking oil. Also, research indicates that the more the mushroom is heated, the less effective its anti-obesity activity. To summarize, the best way to consume maitake is to eat the whole mushroom, including the cooking liquids, and to be careful not to overcook it.

MAITAKE TABLETS

Most people will find maitake supplements as capsules, caplets and liquid extracts more convenient to take. Since there are several varieties of maitake, make sure it is *Grifola frondosa*, the most potent of all.

Maitake caplets consist of the whole, concentrated and dried mushroom powder and are recommended as a tonic or adaptogen (regulating blood pressure, blood sugar, cholesterol, body weight, etc.). The usual recommendation is one to two grams (1,000–2,000 mg) daily for preventive purposes, or three to five grams therapeutically, preferably between or before meals.

THE "ONE-AND-ONLY" D-FRACTION

Use maitake D-fraction (capsules or liquid), the optimum extract of beta glucans, for extra immune support. D-fraction is now the basis of all research in the area of immune-related diseases (colds to cancer). Don't be misled by other products claiming similar effects as D-fraction. Consumers should use extreme caution with a product supported by only one researcher. I always have some reservations when I see such products because the researcher usually maintains some vested interest in the product or the company that manufactures it. I know there are a few of such mushroom-based products in the U.S. market. D-fraction has been the basis of a number of studies conducted by several independent researchers. It is the only standardized extract that has been on the market for ten years. D-fraction has been used by thousands of health professionals and is the product of choice for clinical and laboratory studies with FDA approval for an IND trial. Other products could only claim anecdotal stories, if any.

Take six mg (about six drops) of D-fraction two or three times daily. Therapeutic doses have been as high as 30–100 mg/day (30–100 drops). For best results, use D-fraction along with vitamin C supplements. Vitamin C helps break up large molecular weights of maitake, thus enhancing absorption. Vitamin C is also essential for white blood cells.

TEAS

As a beverage, drink maitake tea, which is available combined with complementary herbs such as green tea and Siberian ginseng. All products are available through natural food and supplement stores.

References

1. Hamaguchi, A. et al, "The Chemical Structure of an Antitumor Polysaccharide in Fruit Bodies of Grifola frondosa (Maitake)," Chem Pharm Bull, 35(3), 1162-1168, 1987.
2. Adachi, K., et al, "Potentiation of Host-Mediated Antitumor Activity in Mice by Beta-Glucan obtained from Grifola Frondosa (Maitake)," Chem Pharm Bull, 35(1), 262-270) 1987.
3. Babal, K. "The Cancer-Fighting Qualities of Mushrooms," Nutrition Science News, 2(3), 141-2, 1997.
4. Hishida, I., et al, "Antitumor Activity Exhibited by Orally Administered Extract from Fruit Body of Grifola frondosa (Maitake)," Chem Pharm Bull, 36(5) 1819-1827, 1988.
5. Lieberman, S. and Babal, K. "Maitake: King of Mushrooms," Keats Publishing, New Canaan, Connecticut, 1997, p.17.
6. Lieberman, S. and Babal, K. ibid., p.18.
7. Shirota, M. "What You Should Know About Medicinal Mushrooms", Explore, 7(2), 48-52, 1996.
8. Jones, K. "Maitake: A Potent Medicinal Food," Alternative and Complimentary Therapies, Dec. 1998.
9. Tazaki, H., et al, "Induction of Apoptosis in Human Prostatic Cancer Cells with B-Glucan (Maitake Mushroom Polysaccharide," Molecular Biology, Vol. 4, No. 1, 7-13, 2000.
10. Maitake Products, Inc. Ridgefield Park, New Jersey, (800) 747-7418, www.MAITAKE.com.
11. In-Vitro Anti-HIV Drug Screening Results, Developmental Therapeutics Program, National Cancer Institute, Jan 17, 1992 (Unpublished).
12. Kubo, K., et al "Anti-Diabetic Activity Present in Fruit Body of Grifola frondosa (Maitake)," Biol Pharm Bull, 17(8) 1106-10 1994.
13. Kubo, K., et al "Anti-Diabetic Mechanism of Maitake (Grifola frondosa)", Mushroom Biology and Mushroom Products, Penn State Univ, ISBN, 215-222, 1996.
14. Adachi, K., et al, "Blood Pressure-Lowering Activity Present in the Fruit Body of Grifola frondosa (Maitake)," Chem Pharm Bull, 36(3), 1000-1006, 1988.
15. Kimura, K., et al, "Effects of Shiitake and Maitake on Plasma Cholesterol and Blood Pressure," Medicinal Effects of Edible Mushrooms, Tohoku Univ & Mushroom Institute of Japan, 1-10, Mar 1988.
16. Ohtsuru, M., "Anti-Obesity Activity Exhibited by Orally Administered Powder of Maitake (Grifola frondosa)," Anshin, 188-200, July 1992.
17. Yokota, M., "Observatory Trial of Anti-Obesity Activity of Maitake (Grifola frondosa)," Anshin, 202-204, July 1992.
18. Preuss, H., et al, "Effects of Maitake Mushroom and Two Extracts on Blood Pressure (BP) and Other Parameters in 2 Rat Strains," J Am Coll Nutr, 17:507, 1998.
19. Cichoke, A., "Maitake: The King of Mushrooms," Townsend Letter for Doctors & Patients, 432-433, May 1994.

About the Authors

Dr. Shari Lieberman earned her Ph.D. in Clinical Nutrition and Exercise Physiology from The Union Institute, Cincinnati, Ohio and her M.S. degree in Nutrition, Food Science and Dietetics from New York University. She is a Certified Nutrition Specialist (CNS), a Fellow of the American College of Nutrition (FACN), a member of the New York Academy of Science and board member of the American Preventive Medical Association. Dr. Lieberman is author of several books, including *Get Off the Menopause Roller Coaster* (Avery 2000), *The Real Vitamin Mineral Book* (Avery 1997) and the soon-to-be-released *Dare to Lose* (Avery, 2001). She is also columnist for *Better Nutrition for Today's Living*. Dr. Lieberman has been in private practice as a clinical nutritionist for more than 20 years in New York City.

Ken Babal is a certified licensed nutritionist through American Health Science University and a member of the Society of Certified Nutritionists. He has a clinical nutrition practice in Los Angeles and is staff nutritionist for Erewhon Natural Foods Market. His articles have appeared in many publications, including *Nutrition Science News*, *Let's Live* and *Health Store News*, and has been quoted in others, including *The Los Angeles Times*. Ken is author of *Good Digestion: Your Key to Vibrant Health* (Alive 2000) and appears in the Discovery Health Channel documentary *Alternatives Uncovered*.

Woodland Health Series

Definitive Natural Health Information At Your Fingertips!

The Woodland Health Series offers a comprehensive array of single topic booklets, covering subjects from fibromyalgia to green tea to acupressure. If you enjoyed this title, look for other WHS titles at your local health-food store, or contact us. Complete and mail (or fax) us the coupon below and receive the complete Woodland catalog and order form—free!

Or . . .

- Call us toll-free at (800) 777-2665
- Visit our website (www.woodlandpublishing.com)
- Fax the coupon (and other correspondence) to (801) 785-8511